D1570856

Taking Control: My Medical Journal

~Two month Journal~

A toolkit for people trying to unravel the mysteries of physical reactions – caused by such things as MCAD, MCAS, Mastocytosis, mast cells, SIBO, IBS, IgE allergies, Histamine Intolerance, Salicylate/Oxalate/food intolerances, etc.

Taking Control: My Medical Journal
Written by
Patty A. Wright

Second Edition 2022
Printed in the United States of America

ISBN: 9798523704017

Cover photography © Patty A. Wright

Personal Information

Name: _____

Address: _____

_____

Cell Phone Number: _____

Work Phone Number: _____

Emergency Contact: _____

Phone Number: _____

Medical I.D. Number: _____

Doctor: _____

Phone Number: _____

Doctor: _____

Phone Number: _____

Medical I.D. Number: _____

Carrier: _____

Dedication

To Rita and Joanna
for being supportive, critical, holding me
accountable, and for always being there
guarding my back as best friends do;

To Jackie and David-
for being the very definition of family.

To my husband Jim –
Soulmate, friend, the one who completes
me.

And to all the patients working diligently
for a better life....

Journal Contents

This journal is not meant to give medical advice or offer a diagnosis. It is merely a tool – an important tool – that will give you the keys to unlock your particular body's unique language and puzzles.

Introduction

We get it.

You feel like your life has been stolen from you. It feels like your body has taken on a life of its own – and it's not bothering to consult you on how it affects your own life.

Having a body that seems to be randomly complicating your life with odd reactions and symptoms that seem to come out of nowhere, with no rhyme or reason, and make you feel like your life is completely out of control.

So you do what any rational person would do: you researched on line and joined Facebook support groups. They told you the solution was simple: Eat . . . an elimination diet . . . a low histamine diet . . . low FODMAP . . . keto . . . paleo . . . . vegetarian . . . vegan . . . organic . . . low FODMAP . . . low oxalate . . . low salicylate . . . failsafe . . . celiac . . . dairy free . . . Gluten free . . . . add probiotics . . . do yoga . . . mindful meditation . . . prayer . . . but most of all . . . exercise . . . just exercise more . . .

STOP

BREATHE

The most important fact to understand is that you are a completely unique individual and both the THINGS that your body reacts to and HOW it reacts will be as unique as you are.

We're going to say that again.

YOU ARE UNIQUE AND COMPLETELY DIFFERENT FROM ANY OTHER PERSON.

Whether you have MCAD, MCAS, SM, HI, SIBO, MCA, IBS, etc., no cookie-cutter diet or environmental solution is going to work for everyone. In addition, your body's reaction may be to something other than the primary "trigger" you've identified – such as the method a food is cooked or stored rather than the food itself. Further complicating matters is that reaction can take up to 48 hours to appear after encountering the trigger.

We know. It sounds unbelievably complicated and overwhelming. The key is to discover your own body's unique language so you can begin listening to it and get control of your life back.

The only way to do that is to journal.

By recording both potential triggers and potential reactions over time can be seen that help you gain control.

The long-standing issue with journaling is that, when using blank notebooks, it can be a messy, complicated task that often ends in nothing more than frustration when trying to determine the meaning of various notes, or worse, trying to find the various papers you've made those scribbled notes on.

Thus was born this journal.

With clear organization, easy to identify correlations between triggers and reactions - patterns can be seen.

We hope this journal is the key that gives you control once again.

** This journal is not meant to give medical advice or offer a diagnosis. It is merely a tool – an important tool – that will give you the keys to unlock your particular body's unique puzzles. **

How To Use This Journal

NOTE: If you suspect that you have IgE allergies, it is strongly recommended that you receive allergy skin testing from your doctor if you are able to.

This journal is set up with a two-page per day system. The pages are undated, allowing you to use multiple sets a day if needed.

ON THE LEFT PAGE, record the time and possible trigger your body was exposed to. Anything that puts stress on your body can cause a reaction – including, but not limited to:

Food   Sunlight
Hormonal Changes   Exercise
Hot water   Stress
Scents   Sexual Activity
Anesthesia   Insect stings
Barometric changes   Medication
Medication fillers
Extreme emotions (happiness, sadness, etc)
Showers (water pressure)
Make-up/hygiene products
Temperature (hot/cold)
Laundry/cleaning products
Dyes (in food and medication)

NOTE: When recording food, be sure to note cooking and storage method, as well as any spices or additives used.

ON THE RIGHT PAGE, record any possible reactions your body may be having to a trigger. Remember, mast cells initiate these reactions, and because mast cells are in every system and every organ, the symptoms of a reaction can occur throughout your body.

REACTIONS MAY INCLUDE*:

Mouth/Face Symptoms – Itchy, scratchy, tingly, sore mouth, tongue or throat; geographic tongue; mouth sores; coughing; sneezing; runny nose; swollen, itchy, watery, or red eyes; angioedema (swelling of face, eyes, lips); swollen glands; flushing; wheezing; trouble swallowing; esophageal spasms.

Skin Symptoms – Rash, spots, hives, flushing, itching, severe sweating, numbness or tingling, inflammation, unexplained bruising.

GI Symptoms – Nausea, diarrhea, vomiting, GI pain (liver, spleen, bladder, kidney, stomach, intestinal), bloating, constipation, IC (frequent urination), heartburn, gas.

OBGYN Symptoms – Pain; painful, heavy periods; PMS. Endometriosis and adenomyosis are common.

Neurological Symptoms – Headaches, anxiety, vertigo, changes in vision, changes in tinnitus, sudden weakness, brain fog, joint / muscle pain, confusion, aphasia.

Cardiac Symptoms – Sudden drops or rise in blood pressure, racing heartbeat, chest pain, fainting, arrhythmia (irregular heart-beat).

SEE EXAMPLES ON NEXT PAGES

* It is important to remember that these symptoms can also be commonly attributed to other illnesses, diseases, and conditions. Consult your doctor to eliminate these possibilities before assuming they are related to intolerance. This journal is to help identify other possible reasons after these are eliminated.

On this page, note everything that could contain a trigger. Make sure you include brands of medications, ingredients / brands of food, and anything pertinent during all activities.

EXAMPLE

Day: Monday   **Date:** March 1, 2019

Time:	Medication, Foods, Activities (Possible Triggers)
7:30 am	2 Boiled COC pasteurized eggs 1 pc Panera sourdough bread Kerrygold grass-fed butter
8:00 am	CVS brand ratididne 1.50 mg CVS brand certrizine 10 mg Ketotifen sawaii 10 mg
8:30 am	10 min shower, hot water Dove white bar soap Aussie Mega moist shampoo, 3 min miracle conditioner - moist
12:30 pm 12:50 pm	Drive to . . . Shopping at Joanne's (Cinnamon pine cones in entrance)
1:00 pm	CBS brand liquid dye free Benadryl, cherry flavor
5:00 pm	Poland Spring bottled water Rotisserie chicken stop and shop Iceberg lettuce, olive oil, Garlic salt, oregano, fresh ground pepper

On this page, note anything that could possibly be a reaction . . . . even if it later turns out to be not a reaction, it is best to note everything to be safe.

EXAMPLE

Day: Monday   **Date:** March 1, 2019

Time:	Symptoms	BP
7:30 am		84/110
8:45 am	Over-all body rash, flushing, exhaustion, tacacardia	
12:55 pm	Instant diarrhea	98/175
1:20 pm		90/130

At least nightly review reactions and reference back to determine the possible trigger that caused it.

Highlight or circle the two, and draw lines between the two – or more, if possible triggers are multiple. Remember, especially with food, the trigger can be up to 48 hours earlier.

With food reactions, remember the following:

- Reactions can be to additives in purchased food.
- Reactions can be to the spices, oils, or additives used in the preparation or cooking process.
- If you are reacting to histamine, the following raise histamine in foods and can cause "safe" foods to become "unsafe":
    o Method of cooking
    o Age of meat
    o Storage: leftovers / buffets

At the end of the week, make notes in the "Weekly Summary" of what you felt you had reactions to, and what the reactions were.

When you are sure you had a particular reaction to something, note it at the beginning under "known triggers". This will help both you and your doctor. It's easy to remember you were triggered by something, yet easy to forget what the reaction was.

As time goes along, your list of things your body reacts to may indicate a "global" issue with a category of things. Identifying a category of things your body doesn't tolerate can help you quickly eliminate possible issues and understand what seem like "odd" reactions – such as a reaction to all tree nuts, except cashews.

Common categories are:

- If you react to chocolate, licorice, canned tuna:
  - You may have a nickel allergy. See page 167.

- If you react to aspirin, quercetin, some nuts, some apples, lettuce except iceberg, cinnamon, coconut, mint:
  - You may have a salicylate intolerance. See page 164

- If you react to leftovers, buffets, avocado, citrus, fermented foods, red wine, vinegar containing foods:
  - You may have a histamine intolerance. See page 158.

- If you react to beer, berries, legumes, citrus:
  - You may have an oxalate intolerance. See page 169.

- If you react to apple, celery, kiwi, melons, papaya:
  - You may have a latex allergy. See page 162.

- If you react to raw fruits and vegetables, with mouth and throat reactions – sores, burning, itching, geographic tongue:
  - You may have Oral Allergy Syndrome. See page 163.

AN IMPORTANT NOTE ABOUT THE "BUCKET"

You've probably heard the terms "emptying the bucket" or "my bucket is full".

This refers to a "build up" of mild reactions until mast cells degranulate because they can't control the reactions any longer.

Using the metaphor of a bucket helps to illustrate that a person can be having mild reactions, perhaps without noticing or treating them, so the mast cells are calmed down in between reactions.

MAST CELL ACTIVATION DISEASE (SYNDROME etc) OR HISTAMINE INTOLERANCE?

This is a common question.

Histamine Intolerance occurs when your body is unable to process and rid itself of histamine.

Your body encounters histamines when you eat high histamine foods, or when your mast cells try to protect you from an intruder and release histamine and 200+ other chemicals (mediators.)

Mast Cells are the leaders of the immune system. They are in all the organs and tissues to detect when you encounter a wound, bacteria, allergen, or stressor. When detected, they can "leak" appropriate chemicals or completely degranulate (explode) and release all 200+ chemicals.

Odd reactions to stress, emotions, showers, heat, allergens you do not have an IgE allergy to... are a malfunction of your mast cells and diagnostic of a MCAD.

A person can have just a Mast Cell Activation Disease and appropriately process and rid the body of the histamines released. This would still give one the symptoms of a reaction.

A person can also have both a Mast Cell Activation Disease AND Histamine Intolerance. This generally results in the reactions lasting longer due to the body's inability to process the histamines released.

This can result in a second type of "Bucket" – that of histamines building up that are not yet processed out. A full "histamine bucket" can lead to longer and stronger reactions to actual allergies and stress.

However, a person with JUST Histamine Intolerance would never have reactions to things they do not have an IgE allergy to, or to minor stresses – as properly acting mast cells would not release their histamines and other chemicals to protect the body when there is no actual threat, or the threat does not warrant a major reaction (such as exposure to sun, a small cut, normal emotions and exercise, etc.)

Yes, it's yet another puzzle piece to figure out. This journal should point to which it is.

AN IMPORTANT NOTE ABOUT ANAPHALAXIS

Contrary to what most people believe, anaphylaxis does not always come on as an instant GRADE 4 anaphylactic shock, which most people are familiar with when peanuts and bee stings are involved.

There are 5 Grades of anaphylaxis that everyone whose bodies experience multiple allergic type reactions should be aware of. It can present with non-life-threatening symptoms that precede and can develop into life-threatening symptoms.

Anaphylaxis is a serious, life-threatening systemic reaction. It is possible to be in an extended, long-term anaphylaxis Grade 1, 2, or 3, without progressing to Grade 4 or 5 – but your body is still in crisis and the anaphylaxis needs to be dealt with effectively to protect your body and your safety.

Rescue meds are important in Grades 2 & 3 to prevent Grade 4 & 5, and a plan should be discussed and agreed upon with your doctor.

ANAPHYLAXIS
(Ring and Messmer - and

GRADE 1	GRADE 2
Symptoms in one organ system	Symptoms in more than one organ system
Skin – Itching, uticaria, flushing, sensations of warmth, angioedema	**Skin** – Itching, uticaria, flushing, sensations of warmth, angioedema
GI Tract – Itchy throat, cough, nausea, metallic taste	**Abdomen** – Vomiting, diarrhea
Conjunctival – Watery eyes, itchiness, redness	**Upper respiratory** – Sneezing, congestion, nasal itchiness, runny nose
Neurological – Headache, feeling of impending doom, behavior changes	**Lower respiratory** – Asthma, cough, wheezing (responds to inhaler)
	Gastrointestinal – Abdominal cramps, vomiting, diarrhea
	Cardiovascular – Tachycardia, hypotension, arrhythmia
	Neurological – Feeling of impending doom, behavior changes,

GRADES
World Allergy Organization Charts)

GRADE 3	GRADE 4
Skin – Itching, uticaria, flushing, sensations of warmth, angioedema	**Skin** – Itching, uticaria, flushing, sensations of warmth, angioedema
Abdomen – Vomiting, diarrhea	**Abdomen** – Vomiting, diarrhea
Lower respiratory – Throat swelling, bronchospasm; asthma not responding to inhaler	**Lower or upper respiratory** – Respiratory failure with or without loss of consciousness
Upper respiratory – Tongue swelling	**Cardiovascular** – Cardiac arrest, shock
Other – Feeling of impending doom, behavior changes	**Other** – Feeling of impending doom, behavior changes

A "SAFE" START?

Many people request an "expected safe place" to start with. Here are some guidelines to choose your start:

EAT FRESH, unprocessed basic food right from the source. The more processed a food, the more additives and preservatives are likely to be in the food.

EAT CLEAN.

A key basis for any diet that seeks to eliminate possible triggers is to choose food and processed food that is closest to the basic food as possible. You can choose ice cream with 25 ingredients – most of them unpronounceable – or one with 4 ingredients. The one with milk, cream, sugar, and vanilla would be the "clean" one. Eating clean eliminates possible reactions to additives rather than the actual food. Fortunately, this diet choice is catching on commercially, so it's easier to obtain "clean" processed food at your local grocery. From a nationwide soup restaurant, to manufacturers of boxed desert mixes, you should be able to find "clean" or "original recipe" products to meet your needs.

FRUITS AND VEGETABLES:

Whether "traditional" or "organic", the fruits and vegetables in your local grocery have pesticides and fertilizers sprayed on them that must be vigorously washed off to prevent reactions that aren't necessarily to the product themselves.

In addition, the product had to be harvested, packed, trucked, packed, sorted, trucked again, and unpacked to reach your local grocery. Even if local products, ripening and mold can cause reactions that aren't necessarily to the food itself.

Farm stands are an option that usually provide these items same day they are picked, if you plan to use them as soon as you get home.

Frozen options are also a good choice – they are professionally washed and flash-frozen immediately after being picked, providing the cleanest, freshest product and highest in nutritional value.

"SAFE" LIST

It is important to remember that each person's body is unique and just because many people don't react to something does not at all mean that you won't react.

With that understanding, the most common "safe foods" are:

Chicken, skinless (not fried)
Beef, especially grass fed
Turkey
White potatoes
White rice
Eggs (raw egg whites are high histamine)
Brussel sprouts
Green beans
Cabbage
Iceberg lettuce
Celery
Oatmeal
Pears
Sugar – white and brown
Cheese – non-aged (cream cheese, cottage
        cheese, feta, ricotta}

My Safe List

My Safe List

My Safe List

My Safe List

My Known Triggers

Date	Trigger - symptoms

My Known Triggers

Date	Trigger - symptoms

My Known Triggers

Date	Trigger - symptoms

My Known Triggers

Date	Trigger - symptoms

My Known Triggers

Date	Trigger - symptoms

My Journal

Day: _____ Date: _____

Time:	Medication, Foods, Activities (Possible Triggers)

Day: _____ Date: _____

Time:	Symptoms	BP

My Journal

Day: _____   Date: _____

Time:	Medication, Foods, Activities (Possible Triggers)

Day: _____ Date: _____

Time:	Symptoms	BP

My Journal

Day: _____ Date: _____

Time:	Medication, Foods, Activities (Possible Triggers)

Day: _____ Date: _____

Time:	Symptoms	BP

My Journal

Day: _____ Date: _____

Time:	Medication, Foods, Activities (Possible Triggers)

Day: _____ Date: _____

Time:	Symptoms	BP

My Journal

Day: _____   Date: _____

Time:	Medication, Foods, Activities (Possible Triggers)

Day: _____ Date: _____

Time:	Symptoms	BP

My Journal

Day: _____   Date: _____

Time:	Medication, Foods, Activities (Possible Triggers)

Day: _____ Date: _____

Time:	Symptoms	BP

My Journal

Day: _____ Date: _____

Time:	Medication, Foods, Activities (Possible Triggers)

Day: _____ Date: _____

Time:	Symptoms	BP

Weekly

Summary

My Journal

Day: _____   Date: _____

Time:	Medication, Foods, Activities (Possible Triggers)

Day: _____ Date: _____

Time:	Symptoms	BP

My Journal

Day: _____   Date: _____

Time:	Medication, Foods, Activities (Possible Triggers)

Day: _____ Date: _____

Time:	Symptoms	BP

My Journal

Day: _____   Date: _____

Time:	Medication, Foods, Activities (Possible Triggers)

Day: _____ Date: _____

Time:	Symptoms	BP

My Journal

Day: _____ Date: _____

Time:	Medication, Foods, Activities (Possible Triggers)

Day: _____ Date: _____

Time:	Symptoms	BP

My Journal

Day: _____ Date: _____

Time:	Medication, Foods, Activities (Possible Triggers)

Day: _____ Date: _____

Time:	Symptoms	BP

My Journal

Day: _____ Date: _____

Time:	Medication, Foods, Activities (Possible Triggers)

Day: _____ Date: _____

Time:	Symptoms	BP

My Journal

Day: _____ Date: _____

Time:	Medication, Foods, Activities (Possible Triggers)

Day: _____ Date: _____

Time:	Symptoms	BP

Weekly

Summary

My Journal

Day: _____   Date: _____

Time:	Medication, Foods, Activities (Possible Triggers)

Day: _____ Date: _____

Time:	Symptoms	BP

My Journal

Day: _____   Date: _____

Time:	Medication, Foods, Activities (Possible Triggers)

Day: _____ Date: _____

Time:	Symptoms	BP

My Journal

Day: _____ Date: _____

Time:	Medication, Foods, Activities (Possible Triggers)

Day: _____ Date: _____

Time:	Symptoms	BP

My Journal

Day: _____   Date: _____

Time:	Medication, Foods, Activities (Possible Triggers)

Day: _____ Date: _____

Time:	Symptoms	BP

My Journal

Day: _____   Date: _____

Time:	Medication, Foods, Activities (Possible Triggers)

Day: _____ Date: _____

Time:	Symptoms	BP

My Journal

Day: _____ Date: _____

Time:	Medication, Foods, Activities (Possible Triggers)

Day: _____ Date: _____

Time:	Symptoms	BP

My Journal

Day: _____   Date: _____

Time:	Medication, Foods, Activities (Possible Triggers)

Day: _____   Date: _____

Time:	Symptoms	BP

Weekly

Summary

My Journal

Day: _____ Date: _____

Time:	Medication, Foods, Activities (Possible Triggers)

Day: _____ Date: _____

Time:	Symptoms	BP

My Journal

Day: _____ Date: _____

Time:	Medication, Foods, Activities (Possible Triggers)

Day: _____ Date: _____

Time:	Symptoms	BP

My Journal

Day: _____   Date: _____

Time:	Medication, Foods, Activities (Possible Triggers)

Day: _____ Date: _____

Time:	Symptoms	BP

My Journal

Day: _____ Date: _____

Time:	Medication, Foods, Activities (Possible Triggers)

Day: _____ Date: _____

Time:	Symptoms	BP

My Journal

Day: _____ Date: _____

Time:	Medication, Foods, Activities (Possible Triggers)

Day: _____ Date: _____

Time:	Symptoms	BP

My Journal

Day: _____ Date: _____

Time:	Medication, Foods, Activities (Possible Triggers)

Day: _____ Date: _____

Time:	Symptoms	BP

My Journal

Day: _____   Date: _____

Time:	Medication, Foods, Activities (Possible Triggers)

Day: _____ Date: _____

Time:	Symptoms	BP

Weekly

Summary

My Journal

Day: _____ Date: _____

Time:	Medication, Foods, Activities (Possible Triggers)

Day: _____ Date: _____

Time:	Symptoms	BP

My Journal

Day: _____   Date: _____

Time:	Medication, Foods, Activities (Possible Triggers)

Day: _____ Date: _____

Time:	Symptoms	BP

My Journal

Day: _____   Date: _____

Time:	Medication, Foods, Activities (Possible Triggers)

Day: _____ Date: _____

Time:	Symptoms	BP

My Journal

Day: _____   Date: _____

Time:	Medication, Foods, Activities (Possible Triggers)

Day: _____   Date: _____

Time:	Symptoms	BP

My Journal

Day: _____ Date: _____

Time:	Medication, Foods, Activities (Possible Triggers)

Day: _____ Date: _____

Time:	Symptoms	BP

My Journal

Day: _____ Date: _____

Time:	Medication, Foods, Activities (Possible Triggers)

Day: _____ Date: _____

Time:	Symptoms	BP

My Journal

Day: _____ Date: _____

Time:	Medication, Foods, Activities (Possible Triggers)

Day: _____ Date: _____

Time:	Symptoms	BP

Weekly

Summary

My Journal

Day: _____ Date: _____

Time:	Medication, Foods, Activities (Possible Triggers)

Day: _____ Date: _____

Time:	Symptoms	BP

My Journal

Day: _____   Date: _____

Time:	Medication, Foods, Activities (Possible Triggers)

Day: _____ Date: _____

Time:	Symptoms	BP

My Journal

Day: _____   Date: _____

Time:	Medication, Foods, Activities (Possible Triggers)

Day: _____ Date: _____

Time:	Symptoms	BP

My Journal

Day: _____ Date: _____

Time:	Medication, Foods, Activities (Possible Triggers)

Day: _____ Date: _____

Time:	Symptoms	BP

My Journal

Day: _____ Date: _____

Time:	Medication, Foods, Activities (Possible Triggers)

Day: _____ Date: _____

Time:	Symptoms	BP

My Journal

Day: _____ Date: _____

Time:	Medication, Foods, Activities (Possible Triggers)

Day: _____ Date: _____

Time:	Symptoms	BP

My Journal

Day: _____ Date: _____

Time:	Medication, Foods, Activities (Possible Triggers)

Day: _____ Date: _____

Time:	Symptoms	BP

Weekly

Summary

My Journal

Day: _____ Date: _____

Time:	Medication, Foods, Activities (Possible Triggers)

Day: _____ Date: _____

Time:	Symptoms	BP

My Journal

Day: _____ Date: _____

Time:	Medication, Foods, Activities (Possible Triggers)

Day: _____ Date: _____

Time:	Symptoms	BP

My Journal

Day: _____ Date: _____

Time:	Medication, Foods, Activities (Possible Triggers)

Day: _____ Date: _____

Time:	Symptoms	BP

My Journal

Day: _____ Date: _____

Time:	Medication, Foods, Activities (Possible Triggers)

Day: _____ Date: _____

Time:	Symptoms	BP

My Journal

Day: _____ Date: _____

Time:	Medication, Foods, Activities (Possible Triggers)

Day: _____ Date: _____

Time:	Symptoms	BP

My Journal

Day: _____   Date: _____

Time:	Medication, Foods, Activities (Possible Triggers)

Day: _____ Date: _____

Time:	Symptoms	BP

My Journal

Day: _____   Date: _____

Time:	Medication, Foods, Activities (Possible Triggers)

Day: _____ Date: _____

Time:	Symptoms	BP

Weekly

Summary

My Journal

Day: _____ Date: _____

Time:	Medication, Foods, Activities (Possible Triggers)

Day: _____ Date: _____

Time:	Symptoms	BP

My Journal

Day: _____   Date: _____

Time:	Medication, Foods, Activities (Possible Triggers)

Day: _____ Date: _____

Time:	Symptoms	BP

My Journal

Day: _____   Date: _____

Time:	Medication, Foods, Activities (Possible Triggers)

Day: _____ Date: _____

Time:	Symptoms	BP

My Journal

Day: _____ Date: _____

Time:	Medication, Foods, Activities (Possible Triggers)

Day: _____ Date: _____

Time:	Symptoms	BP

My Journal

Day: _____   Date: _____

Time:	Medication, Foods, Activities (Possible Triggers)

Day: _____ Date: _____

Time:	Symptoms	BP

My Journal

Day: _____   Date: _____

Time:	Medication, Foods, Activities (Possible Triggers)

Day: _____ Date: _____

Time:	Symptoms	BP

My Journal

Day: _____   Date: _____

Time:	Medication, Foods, Activities (Possible Triggers)

Day: _____ Date: _____

Time:	Symptoms	BP

Weekly

Summary

Histamine in Foods

We know you've done research – so you already know the "histamine in foods lists" contradict each other widely.

There are a few agreed on items:

Aged foods – Foods build histamine as they age. That means older food contains more histamine. This includes – leftovers, processed / cured / smoked meats, buffets, slow-cooked foods (crock pots, baking, frying), aged cheese, refrigerated meats and fish.

Fermented foods – Alcohol (especially red wine, beer), sauerkraut, soy sauce, yogurt, kefir (drinkable yogurt).

Vinegar / Vinegar containing foods – Salad dressing, mayonnaise, pickled beets, ketchup, chili sauce, pickles, relishes, olives, coleslaw, prepared mustard.

In addition, the following foods are agreed as being high in histamine by 4 or more available "lists". That doesn't mean that will necessarily be your personal experience.

Beverages – Coffee, tea (black and green), alcohol

Food additives – Artificial sweeteners, artificial colors / flavors (often a trigger in medicines), BHA, BHT

Fruits – Cherries, cranberries, currents, dates / figs, loganberries, peaches, pumpkins, prunes, plums, raisins, grapes, raspberries, tomatoes, avocados – and all products made using these fruits (jams, jellies, juices)

Legumes – Peanuts, soy, lentils, beans – and all products, butters, and oils made with these, such as tofu, hummus, and "vegetable oil" (usually soybean oil).

Tree nuts – Cashews, walnuts, Brazil nuts, macadamia nuts

Spices – Chili powder, cinnamon, cayenne, cloves, anise, nutmeg, curry powder.

Vegetables – Spinach, eggplant, mushrooms, avocados, tomatoes

Histamine Liberators

While the following foods do not contain high amounts of histamine themselves, they cause the body to release histamine.

If you do not normally react to these foods, but you are suffering from allergy symptoms (such as hay fever) or another type of histamine flare, it's generally recommended you avoid these foods.

- Cocoa and chocolate

- All citrus fruits – oranges, lemons, lime, grapefruit, tangerines, tangelos

- Green cabbage

- Raw egg whites, fish, and shellfish

- Papaya, pineapple, strawberries, tomatoes, ripe bananas

- Additives, including benzoate, nitrites, sulfites, glutamate, food dyes

Low Histamine Foods

Again, these foods were agreed on by at least 4 different lists – but that does not guarantee the histamine level in any food, nor does it guarantee a particular person's body's reaction or non-reaction to it.

Dairy – Raw milk from grass-fed cows, butter (try "Kerry Gold" from grass-fed cows), cream, whey, cream cheese, mozzarella, curd cheese, cottage cheese, mascarpone, ricotta, young Gouda

Fruits – Apples, apricots, bananas with green on them, blackberries, blueberries, cherries, cranberries, currents, lychee, mango, melons, persimmon, watermelon

Protein – Eggs, poultry, pork, venison, etc. – either fresh-butchered or cooked from frozen. Fresh caught fish.

Spices – Table salt, garlic

Sweeteners – Agave syrup, honey, white sugar, brown sugar, stevia

Starches and Grains – Potatoes, sweet potatoes, corn, rice, semolina, wheat flour, pasta

Vegetables – Asparagus, carrots, cauliflower, chicory, cucumber, beetroot, broccoli, iceberg lettuce, leek, onions, paprika, sweet peppers, radishes, rhubarb, zucchini

Latex Cross Reactions

If you have an IgE allergy to latex, you may react to:

Apples, avocado, bananas, carrots, celery, chestnuts, kiwi, melons, papaya, potatoes, tomatoes, melons

Oral Allergy Syndrome

OAS is caused by your immune system recognizing similar proteins in food as the pollen you are allergic to, which causes an allergic response.

This typically occurs in people who have been eating the offending fruit or vegetable for years without an issue. The allergic response usually comes in the form of mouth and throat symptoms – itchiness, swelling, sores, pain.

The allergic response generally only occurs to the raw fruits and vegetables, as cooking destroys the proteins the body is reacting to.

Birch / Adler – Apples, almonds, carrots, celery, cherries, hazelnuts, kiwi, parsley, soybeans

Ragweed Pollen – Bananas, cucumber, melons, zucchini

Grass Pollen – Celery, melons, oranges, peaches, tomatoes, dates, figs, kiwi, peas, potatoes, peanuts

Salicylate Food List

Unlike histamine, there appears to be almost a universal agreement on which foods and medicines are high in salicylates – the main ingredient in aspirin. However, this list was compiled from a minimum of 4 sources that agreed.

That does not mean the list is complete and finite, nor does it guarantee a particular person's body's reaction or non-reaction.

Foods High in Salicylates

Beverages – Alcohol (especially red wine), coffee, birch beer, root beer, carbonated drinks, water "enhanced with minerals", rice milk, soy milk

Fruits – Apples (except Granny Smith), apricot, avocado, blackberries, blackcurrant berries, blueberries, boysenberries, cranberries, huckleberries, gooseberries, loganberries, mulberries, raspberries, strawberries, youngberries, oranges, lemons, tangelo, grapefruit, mandarins, cherries, currants, dates, prunes, raisins, figs, grapes, guava, kiwi, cantaloupe, honeydew, watermelon, peaches, nectarines, pineapple, plums, tomatoes

Legumes, Nuts, and Seeds – Almonds, Brazil nuts, macadamia nuts, peanuts, pine nuts, pistachio nuts, poppy seeds, sesame seeds

Meat, Fish, and Eggs – Liver and prawns

Oils and Fats – Almond oil, corn oil, coconut oil, olive oil, peanut oil, sesame oil, walnut oil, mayonnaise, margarine

Spices – All-spice, anise seed, basil, bay leaf, cayenne celery chili, cinnamon, cloves, cumin, curry powder, dill, ginger, licorice, mace, all mints, mustard, nutmeg, oregano, paprika, pepper, rosemary, sage, tarragon, turmeric, thyme, wintergreen, Worcestershire sauce

Vegetables – Alfalfa sprouts, artichoke, asparagus, broccoli, broad beans, cauliflower, chili pepper (all colors), chicory, cucumber, endive, okra, olives, peppers, radish, spinach, squash, water chestnut, watercress, zucchini

Additives – Coal tar (often used as the base for commercial vitamins), artificial flavorings, artificial colorings, Azo dyes, Beta hydroxyl acid, VHA, BHT, eucalyptus oils, menthol, red dye (#40), salicylaidehyde, salicylamide, salicylic acid, yellow dye (#5 and #6)

Foods Low in Salicylates

Beverages – Whiskey, gin, vodka

Fruit – Apples (golden and red delicious, Granny Smith), bananas, pears, figs, cherries, grapes, lemons, mango, pawpaw, passion fruit, persimmon, pineapple juice, pomegranate, rhubarb, tamarillo

Vegetables – Green beans, potatoes, peas, tomatoes, Brussel sprouts, cabbage, celery, leek, iceberg lettuce, soybeans, bean sprouts

Legumes, Nuts, and Seeds – Beans, pecans, peanut butter, sesame seeds, hazelnuts, sunflower seeds, cashews, poppy seeds

Seasonings – Garlic, parsley, vinegar, soy sauce, chives, saffron, coriander, salt, horseradish, vanilla

Foods High in Nickel

An allergy to nickel is the most common metal allergy. It can develop at any point in life, and it is life-long.

People who are allergic to nickel and consume it can develop dermatitis ("nickel eczema"), particularly on their hands.

Eating a low nickel diet can assist in helping control the symptoms.

Chocolate / Cocoa

Grains – Bran, buckwheat, millet, muesli, multi-grain breads, oatmeal, rice (unpolished), brown rice, rye bran, wheat, bran, including fiber tablets

Fruit and Berries – Canned fruit, dates, figs, pineapple, prunes, raspberries

Drinks – Chocolate and cocoa drinks, tea and coffee from drink dispensers

Legumes, Nuts, and Seeds – Almonds, cashews, hazelnuts, peanuts, sunflower seeds, sesame seeds

Miscellaneous – Baking powder (in large amounts), licorice, vitamins containing nickel

Vegetables – Canned vegetables, beans (green, brown, white, red kidney), bean sprouts, kale, leeks, lettuce, lentils, peas, spinach, onion, garlic

Meat, Fish, and Poultry – Canned meat and fish, such as tuna, herring, shellfish, salmon, and mackerel; shellfish, such as shrimp, mussels, and crawfish

Also Avoid – Cooking in nickel-plated pans with nickel-plated utensils. Acidic food should not be cooked in stainless steel.

A Note of Hope – High doses of vitamin C or iron can reduce the absorption of nickel. Always check with your doctor before trying supplements.

Foods High in Oxalate

People who have kidney stones, gout, or do not absorb fat well typically need to follow a low oxalate diet.

Fruit – Raspberries, strawberries, blackberries, blueberries, dewberries, gooseberries, kiwi, figs, grapes, currants, lemon, lime, oranges, tangerines, tomatoes

Vegetables – Beans (green, snap, waxed), beets, celery, collards, eggplant, kale, leeks, okra, parsnips, peppers, potatoes (white, sweet), rhubarb, rutabagas, spinach, squash, turnip, yams

Legumes, Nuts, and Seeds – Almonds, garbanzo beans, cashews, peanuts, pecans, sunflower seeds, sesame seeds, soy

Grains – Bran flakes, grits, graham flour, oatmeal, quinoa, white corn

Beverages – Beer, larger draft, pilsner, green tea, Ovaltine, chocolate

Seasonings – Cinnamon, ginger, parsley, cocoa.

Made in United States
North Haven, CT
14 October 2022

25452843R00095